Acknowledgements

Thank You Diante, Mekhi and KyLee Spears, my children, my inspiration, my Strength.

Thank You David Cort @realdavidcort
You were the catalyst for everything I had stewing.

KyLee Spears @piece.ks appearing in photos and participating in our practices.
Photos by Diante Spears @diantespears and Mekhi Spears @masterhotstuff
Printed by CreateSpace, An Amazon.com Company

Forward

I have been involved in personal, mental, and physical practices for 27 years. My hope is to make a good first impression so as to be able to readily share my practices with you in the future. When I began writing I had no idea how to go about writing a book. I practiced these things, applying them to my personal thought process toward writing and developing my own style. I am getting a little better every day, sometimes failing, sometimes having success, and always getting better. My way may seem different than others, and not adhere to the normal way books are written, but I am an individual expressing my own flare. I hope this is clear. I would not want to have my way be exactly like any other way. I hold no credentials and claim no expertise.
I do not have many quotes and no scientific references.
Words are empty until filled with experience.
Only personal practice can make my points for me and translate into success for you.

So,
We begin

Chapter 1

BEGIN

Begin by connecting with the "why?" Why do you want or need to develop a healthy lifestyle? If you want to run an OCR, (Obstacle Course Race), ask yourself why. Go deep. Go beyond the trophy and the egotism and find out truly why. When we begin to find our root motivations we begin to develop meaningful and lasting habits that change our lives for the better. I have talked to a lot of people who express that they practice a sport or activity because it makes them feel like they can do anything. Meanwhile, they fail at human relationships and work jobs they hate. This says to me that they are missing something. Truly feeling like I can do anything should mean I feel like I can do better in my personal relationships, I can find work I love, I can control my mental and physical diets and so on. Discovering your root motivations will unlock all of these things. Are you an attention whore? Do you have a chip on your shoulder because your parents didn't see your value? Do you want to be able to play in the yard with your grand babies? Have you reached a health emergency that must be addressed? Is your motivation preventative? Or, do you just want to be able to do fun stuff, injury and stress free? There are many things that must be considered. Do not stop at the trophy. Go beyond these things.

Now we are beginning to know what our motivation is. So let's look at what we can do, what we have to work with, and where we are. What we do today has to align with our current abilities. The ego can really take hold here and steer us toward mental or physical breaks which can only serve to obstruct. We need to be realistic in the now. Become knowledgeable about your current physical and mental state. Do you have injuries? How is your posture? Do you have physical and mental issues that that you believe are hereditary? Many people have physical and mental issues they believe are hereditary that are only hereditary because people in a group tend to carry themselves the same way. They have the same posture, same gait, move the same, same core beliefs, same motivations and speak the same way. And so their bodies and/or minds build up and/or break down the same. Getting in touch with the, "why?" will make you more knowledgeable about your current mental state. Are you injured in any way? Do you have certain triggers that cause you to lose momentum? We often have triggers that go so far back we forget what causes the reaction. Our minds have decided to skip all the wind up and developed an auto pilot. It could be a simple phrase, facial expression, tone of voice, or a song playing. Begin paying attention to your triggers. Engage them. Do not run away from them.

So, now you are just waking up, you have knowledge of your physical and mental self and you want to get cracking. Where to begin? Start with posture, sitting or standing. Proper posture stabilizes the muscles, the bones, and the nerves. With close attention you can feel proper posture. To make it easy, sit in meditation with good meditation posture, straight back, chin pointing forward, palms of hands resting on knees. Breathing into about 3 inches below the navel and 3 inches in. With attention you will be able to pinpoint exactly where you should feel this. Slow, steady, and controlled breathing. Stand up while maintaining breath control. keeping your upper body in the exact position it was in when sitting. The upper body should be exactly the same. The core should be the same. With your chest out and up slightly. So as to have no strain caused. Shoulders relaxed, Imagine your weight is centered 3 inches below your belly button and 3 inches into your core from there. Remember this spot always. The same place you breathe into. You can imagine riding a horse.

A Fat Horse

Feet further apart than shoulder width.

A Skinny Horse

feet closer than shoulder width apart

Or a healthy horse

Feet shoulder width apart

Pointing the toes out slightly or both forward according to your comfort. Knees bent slightly. When performing any physical activity always return to this stance. Proper posture is the foundation to a stable body. Begin trying to move within this framework when doing all things. A stable body eases the mind. A stable mind eases the body.

You can begin to build your own customized triggers with intention. Wake up at the same time every morning and give attention only to yourself for the first half hour. This time can be expanded as you gain stronger focus. When you wake up begin your programming for the day. Do not focus on the stressful things you need to get done but on the good stuff you will get done. You can keep it simple. When I have work lined up that requires precision, I meditate on precision. The results are pretty cool and can be mind blowing. Do not let the stresses of the world help you forget the mind blowing results of intention.

Begin letting small things go, ie: something someone said or did., the person who cut you off, the mistake you or someone else made, jamming your toe on the end table. Many of these things will continue to happen, some of them every day. To spend energy toward something you can't change is futile and harmful to your mental and physical well being. You will find that the more you let go, the more you can let go. It becomes it's own miraculous feat of strength. Do not let stress help you forget the power of letting go. Better awareness will also help avoid mistakes, toe jams, rude people, and stressful traffic situations.

Make your bed before you leave your sleeping quarters. There is a reason military men and women are made to complete this task immediately upon waking. It sets a precedent towards getting things done for the day right off the bat.

Drink two tall glasses of water. This lubricates and revs up your digestive system for the day, immediately hydrates you and takes up room in your belly you might otherwise fill with more than you need or food you shouldn't eat if your goal is a lifetime of fitness. Consider your belly a camel hump and keep it filled with water.

A healthy diet will include fruit, vegetables, and some lean meat. (If you don't eat meat, find a healthy alternative for your protein needs.) Do not fall for the latest fads. For instance, we are being sold, " sugar free" again. This is a fad that has come and gone and is now back. Fruit is ok. I remember a conversation with someone about avocados. This athlete believed avocados were bad for you because of the, "fat free" fad. Now everyone touts avocados as a superfood. I myself do not count calories. The more I eat, the more energy I have, the further I go. No special diet plans. I eat when I'm hungry, sometimes I eat before I'm hungry if I'm engaged in activities I need fuel for and won't have time to stop and eat. I also allow myself to be hungry often. We are lucky enough to live in a place and time where starvation isn't likely. Programming your body not to freak out when you can't eat will help you concentrate on other things. Your body is very smart and will adapt. No stress. If you stress when you eat, your mind begins to associate eating with stress. If you stress about food when not eating you will get the same result, stress when eating.

Remember, "Out of sight, out of mind." If you store your healthy foods in places you can't see them, you will likely forget about them and return to less suitable items. Make frequent trips to the grocery store and keep the food where you can see it. On the counter and out in the open when you open the refrigerator. The great thing about leaving fresh fruits and vegetables on the counter is, it must be eaten and you get to eat healthy food until it's all gone. Leftovers are amazing when they are half an onion, red pepper, mushrooms, cilantro and so on. Very easy to whip up as well. I have found with fresh food, I am always feasting because it must be eaten. Dispose of the belief that fresh food is expensive. It gets expensive when you start buying into the fads. Simplicity my friends. This idea can be applied to many things.

Do not eat sugar after 6:00 PM. Sugar wakes you up and we are trying to wind down at this time. Go to bed early. Wake up early. Daylight gives energy. If you sleep the day away, you will miss out on a huge all natural energy source. Just like in the morning, at night, one half hour before bed, become intent on yourself. Examine your mental and physical state and direct it toward rest. If you can't sleep, don't worry about it. I find that on nights I can't sleep and I just go with it, in the morning I still have a ton of energy. If I fight it and worry, I burn far more energy and I am lethargic and grumpy in the morning.

We have shown a few workouts in Chapter 3 The simple workouts should be adopted by all levels. Far too often we confuse complicated movements with strength. Without a proper foundation even the most beautiful structures will fall.

Chapter 2

FOUNDATION

Build Insight, Build Knowledge, Build Will Power

Build Insight

Insight will not come in the same way for the same reasons to two different people. We must go within ourselves.

You do not have to do things you don't like. Begin finding activities physical and mental, you can enjoy. This is one place you can go deep and examine a root motivation or demotivation. Have you always said, "I hate running?" Is this really true? Or is it something you started saying long ago for reasons you can't remember, and now you're stuck? I saw this in myself when eating bananas. For years I believed bananas would make me throw up. One day I was wondering if this were true. I began examining my memory and I have an unclear memory of me arguing with my aunt as a small child. I was refusing to eat the banana that morning because it was truly making me sick due to an upset stomach. I wondered if this had linked in my mind sickness and stubbornness to bananas so I stubbornly assumed I would be sick if I ate one from then on. So I tried a banana. I love bananas!

It may also turn out that through attention you find some foods actually do disagree with you more than you knew. Writing down what you ate and how you felt may help you find patterns you were unaware of. I find that the body and mind are very good at what they do and with attention writing it down may be unnecessary. Do not ignore the signs.

Don't be afraid to try different things. Even things you loved as a child but abandoned as childish. Playing will keep your mind and body fresh and will raise your chances of finding something you love. As a child you were likely more inclined to explore exactly the things that drew you by personal instinct.

If you're an extrovert, connect or reconnect with people that are out doing things you're interested in. These people will have either already ran into the natural obstacles involved in these endeavors or they will also be beginning and be another perspective toward figuring it out. Tools are easier gained when everyone is focused on the same results. Be sure to maintain the freedom of your own creativity and do not become subverted by the group or a set of strict ideas. Stay open and you will gain and maintain momentum more readily.

If you are an introvert, figure it out on your own. Introverts have the privilege of less distractions. Introverts can also do well with meeting another introvert who would love to share their knowledge or passion with at least one other person. Going out and learning cool things from other introverts or doing cool things with other introverts may also build tools toward dealing with others when the need arises. Dealing with introverts forces you to look deeper and pay closer attention. This will translate well into group settings.

Begin paying close attention to the feelings you get from people, places and things. You can be very excited about your day and end up spending time with people who, complain, cut you down and manipulate your energy. This can bring your energy down or distract you from your intention at that time. You may find yourself in a place where the light, music, conversation, or atmosphere, brings your energy down or distracts you from your intention at that time. You may have a thing in your life or a place you spend a great deal of time that brings your energy down or distracts you that you could rid yourself of.

Build knowledge

If you've been paying attention to yourself, others, and your surroundings, you will notice that the practice cannot help but build personal and interpersonal knowledge. Meeting with people interested in your chosen activities cannot help but build knowledge toward that activity and working with others toward your intent. Combine the two and you begin to pick up situational cues realized in real time and avoid physical and mental confusion allowing you to apply and adapt prior knowledge to real time situations more readily.

Having begun you likely have built up some physical and mental reps. You have noticed how the mental and physical actions needed are becoming easier. The cool thing is, it only gets better. The catch here is that, to gain knowledge, we have to dispose of the belief that we already know. Curiosity about ourselves, others, and situations must be maintained.

Do not automatically take expert's' word for things. The only way to know for sure is to lay your own hands on the thing. This is how we become sold on fads and convinced we couldn't possibly know what is good for us. I find that many experts are expert at selling you something. Be it an idea or a product. Test things out. If it works toward your intent keep it. If it doesn't work abandon it. Notice if you were sold on how well it worked before or after you began trying it. I encourage this practice for this book.

This isn't to say experts hold no value. An true expert has likely forgotten more than you've learned toward a particular endeavor if you're just starting out. And remember, an expert at one thing will not be an expert at everything. Do not get caught up. Keep in mind; a person may be considered an expert, and be considered unethical.

Be aware that many, (not all) experts are introverts and may have anxiety or habits that are not in accordance with what could be considered social grace. Get to know them anyway. Tolerate their nuances. You will gain empathy and knowledge more readily this way. The techniques you develop dealing with eccentric introverts can be applied to dealing with others, and can only lend to the idea that your own eccentricities are ok.
Become a student of yourself, others and real time situations, and you will become an expert on your very own life. This is where value lies. Write things down if you have to but the good stuff, once seen cannot be unseen. Writing it down is almost ignoring it in my opinion. This opinion comes after writing down a whole lot.

Avoid information overload. Too much information can freeze you up and render you ineffective. Get in the practice of laying hands on whatever it is you are curious about in creative ways. Laying hands on a thing is where the value lies. Listen to Spanish music while learning Spanish. Learning Geometry? Play "Eye Spy" with geometric shapes, angles and lines in real time. Practice relationships by interacting with people you meet. Become interested in them and their interests in the moment.

Build Willpower

Get in the habit of finishing small things you start every day. Wash your dish each time you use it. This is very easy to do and very easy to forget to do. Make your bed when you wake up. It sets up a precedent for getting things done. Drink the entire glass of water. If you started a conversation and you find yourself checking out, use that as a cue to check back in. I like to imagine I have big, adjustable ears. When I find myself checking out I imagine pointing my big adjustable ears at the person talking. I don't get frustrated about losing focus. I just use the loss of focus as a cue to focus. This also builds willpower toward not getting easily frustrated with myself.

Begin setting dates. Eliminate the word, "ish" from your mental diet. "Ish" is a word with no substance. In my opinion it's a word that allows slop. Don't use the word "ish" and do not allow it to infect your intent. "Ish" is a bullying word that allows people to hold your time hostage. It is a lack luster word that can only bring about lackluster results.

Find things you find beautiful and or interesting. Examine them as intensely as you can manage for 5 minutes. Engage them deeply. Examine the filled spaces and the empty spaces. When you get good at 5 minutes, bump it up to 10 minutes. When you get good at examining beautiful and or interesting things, examine ugly and or uninteresting things. You may find yourself finding more things beautiful and or interesting than ever before.

I like to work construction. Often in construction when working with others I find myself having to hold something not heavy or not too heavy while in an awkward position. At first it may be very uncomfortable. I tell myself, "I will hold this forever if needed." and my comfort level instantly increases. The object may slip out of place momentarily or even fall completely. I do not get frustrated. I use the mishap as a cue to tell myself, "I will hold this forever if needed." This cuts down on job stress and has helped me learn various ways to hold a position while remaining comfortable.

Meditation is a practice that can build great willpower. You can focus on "No Mind" or "Single Mind." I have a teacher who would say, " Imagine how powerful "Single Mind" could be if you can achieve "No Mind." No mind can be hard to maintain but easy to find. You can witness it when you drive home and not remember the trip because the route is so ingrained, or when your mind goes blank when startled. It can be witnessed in the gap between thoughts. "No mind" can be practiced by waiting for the gap between thoughts, relaxing into it and not getting too excited when you realize it. In "No Mind", stay calm and aware.

"Single Mind" may be easier and can be applied to anything. When you are washing your dish, be totally focused on the task. The water temperature, the way the water feels, the way the dish rag feels, the scent of the leftover food, the way the dish feels. All the sensations involved washing a dish entails.

Hold a phrase, image or word in your mind for 5 minutes at a time. When you get good at 5 minutes, bump it up to 10.

Hang out with people who promote willpower toward your intentions and not those who chip away at it. Or at least, if you must hang out with people who chip away at your willpower, make your intentions and boundaries clear. People not down for your crew will fall off quickly when you are upfront with them.

Of course this will be easier if you have become clear with yourself about your intentions and boundaries .

Chapter 3
PRACTICES

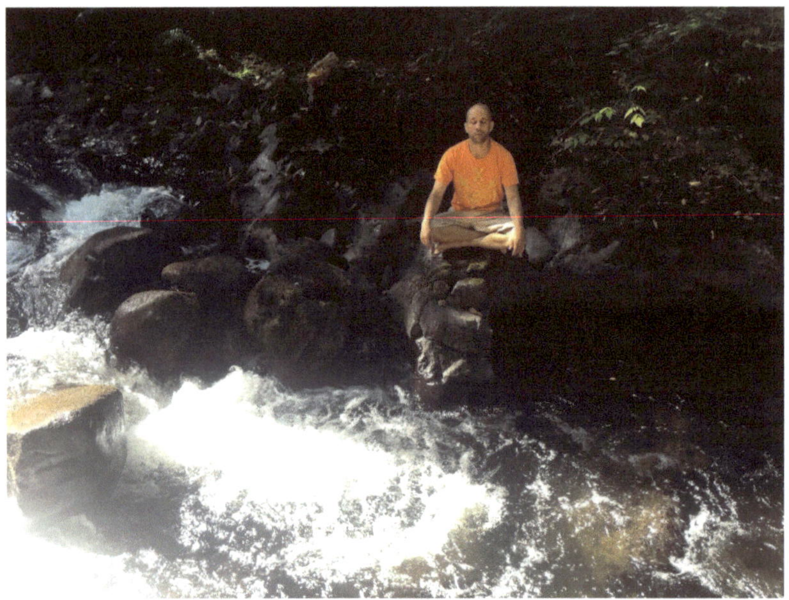

 Upon waking up, assume meditation pose. This can be sitting, standing up, or even lying flat on your back. With practice, staying meditative within movement or restriction can be accomplished. A single pose for reaching a meditative state is not needed however, lying, sitting or standing is a good way to start. Breathe deeply into the area 3 inches below your navel and 3 inches in. If you forget to breathe into this area, use that as a cue to breathe into that area. Feel your weight center in the same spot. If you forget to center your weight in this area, use that as a cue to center your weight in this area. Breathe slow and easy. Keep breathing. If you forget to breathe steady, use that as a cue to breathe steady.

Focus on something. If it's a loved one or loved ones, feel the love. I love my children a great deal and just the thought of them evokes grand feelings. I will picture hugging one of them, all the love I feel, and I will let it wash over me and stay. If it's a course of action, focus on the course of action. This one is easy, I fix something in my head I will do and I go do it. This can be even a small thing like remembering to pick up avocados. Starting small is perfectly fine and remembering how effective little things can be is good practice. If precision is required for the day, focus on precision. Clearly defining the word precision alone will boost your focus toward it immensely. Don't just define the sound of the word. define the feeling it evokes. Ask yourself what precision feels like. If it's a new car, see the new car. If it's the top of a mountain, be on top of the mountain. If it's breath control, just breathe. With practice you will begin to control your breathing more readily, and move on to more complicated breathing techniques. You will be able to use different techniques to hit different gears for each chosen endeavor from washing dishes to running a trail marathon. From flat running, to gearing up for a hill, to making it up the hill, to recovery at the top of the hill, to the float or mad dash downhill depending.

WARM UP

A morning warm up does not have to be long, complicated or stressful.

You can start off before you even sit up from sleep by reaching as far as you can in opposite directions with hands and feet while exhaling deeply. All of your morning stretches can have this same easy feel and be very effective.

After meditating and making your bed, stand up. Find your Horse Stance.

Place your feet shoulder width apart.

Softly bend your knees. Relax all muscles not needed. With practice you will become more familiar with which muscles are needed. Keep your weight evenly distributed between both feet.

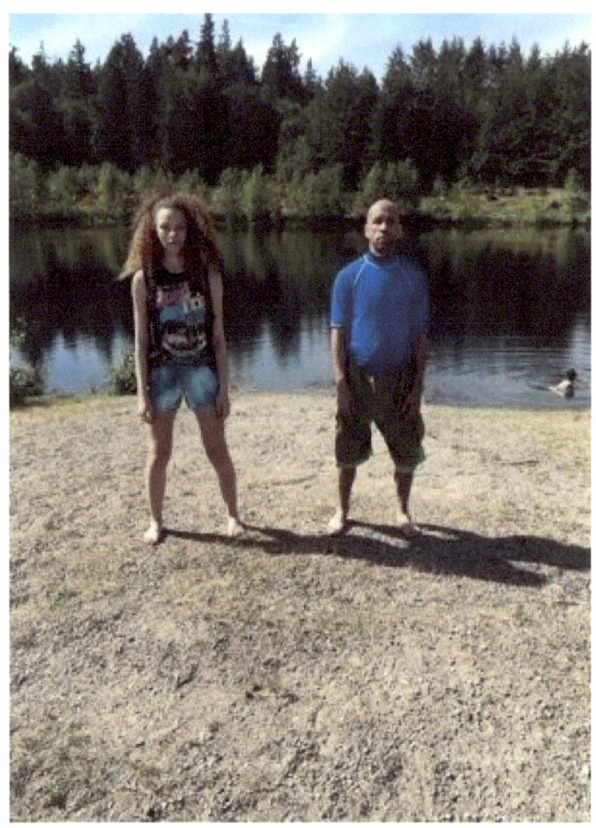

Fat Horse Assume the same position as with Horse Stance but with your feet slightly wider than shoulder width.

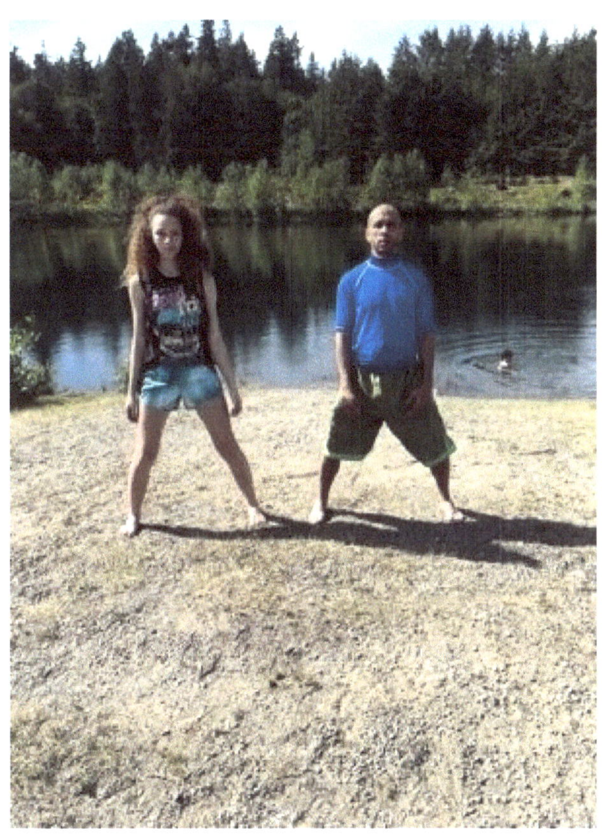

Skinny Horse stance Assume Horse Stance but with feet more narrow than shoulder width.

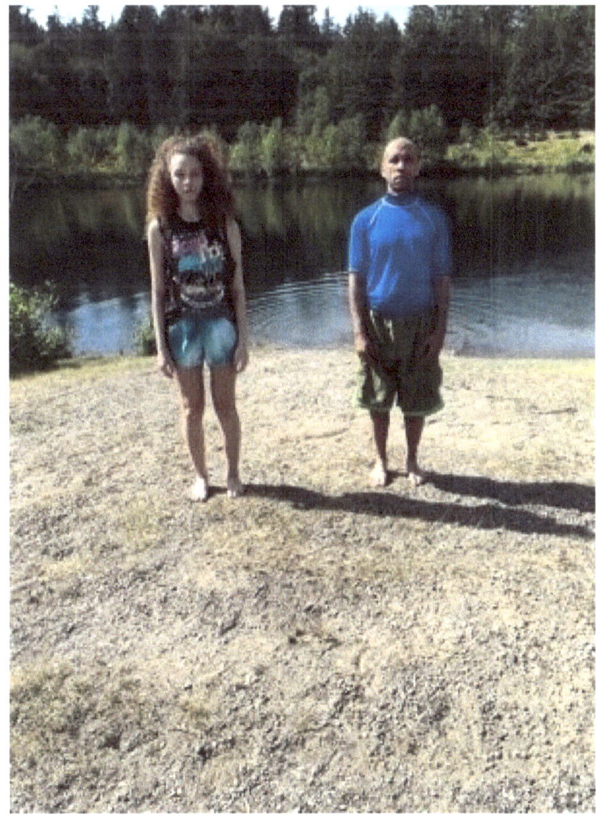

Yes
 Tilt your nose to the floor and to the sky as many times as is comfortable. Pay attention to your spine, your hips and your knees. If these wobble, you are doing it wrong. Nice and easy within a comfortable range of motion.

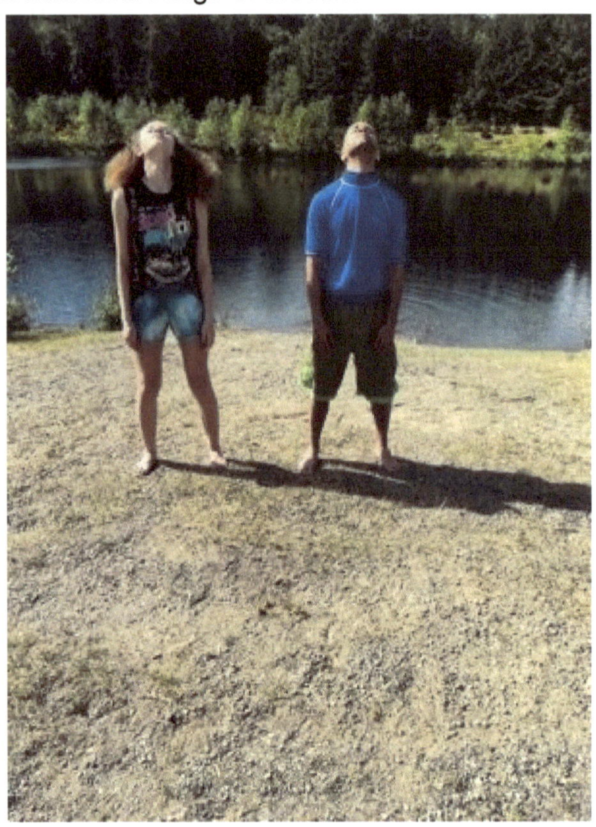

No

Here again, going slow, being intentional, remembering to breathe, remembering where to breathe and where your balance is. Rotate your head slowly and lightly in one direction then the other. The number of times will be determined by how you feel. Go slow however many reps you decide on. Look as far as you can comfortably to the left and then the right for as many times as is comfortable.

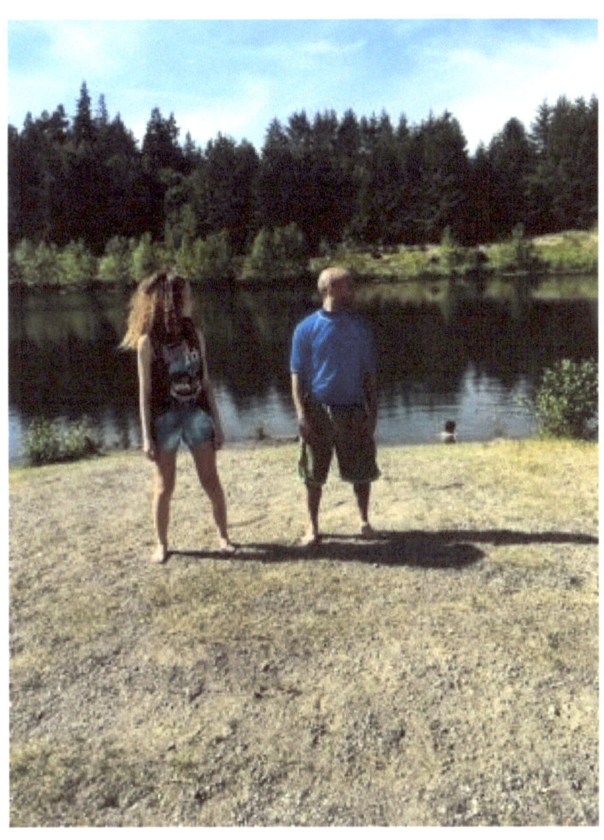

Maybe
Rotate the top of your head in as big of a circle as you can without wobbling your body. Try and keep your neck very relaxed.

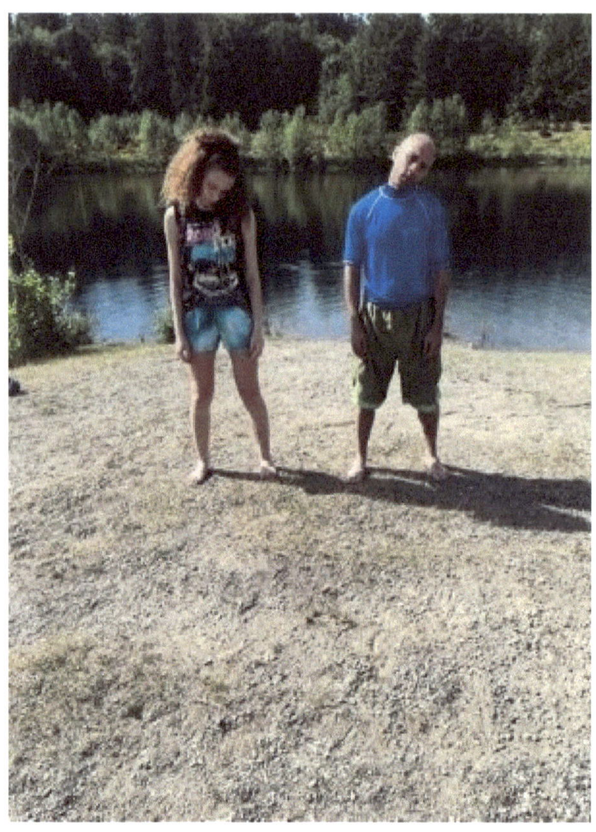

Small arm circles Extend each arm out fully parallel with the ground. Rotate them in small circles forward.

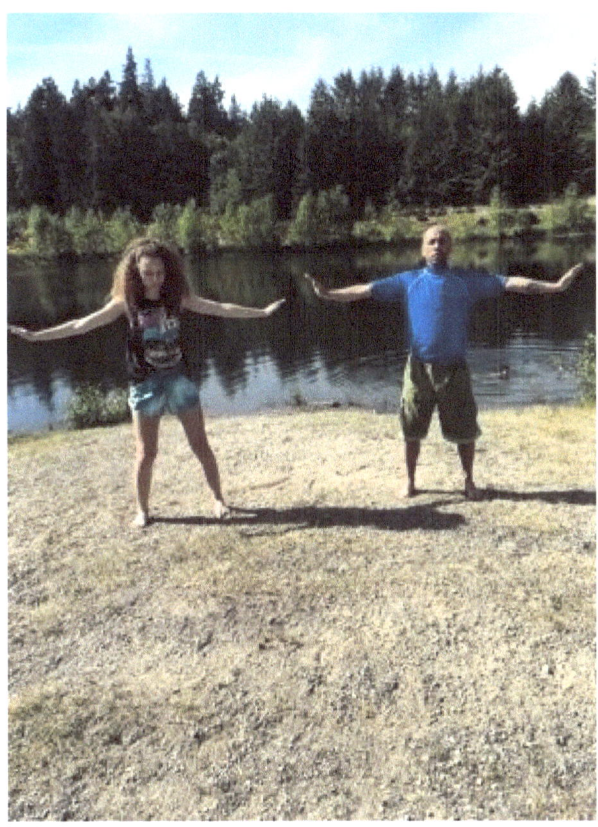

 Pay attention to your body. Make your goal to have no movement in your body other than the rotation of your arms.
No wobble in upper or lower body. Breathing in the same pattern and into the same area we are beginning to find more readily. Do as many as feels comfortable. Now reverse the direction of the circles.
 Shake it out.
 Large Arm Circles Extend Rotate your arms in large circles forward.

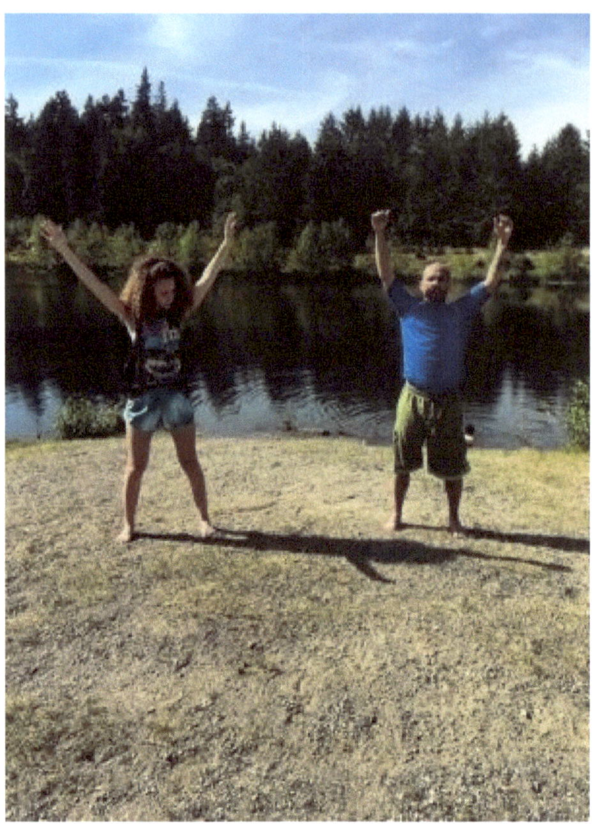

Our goal is to move only our arms while our torso and lower body remain still. Keep good balance and good breathing. Do this as many times as is comfortable. Reverse direction. Shake it out.

Core Rotations
Make both hands into a fist Raise fists and touch each set of knuckles together at your center line or where your chest muscles meet. Keep elbows parallel to the ground. Rotate your torso only keeping fists touching at your center line.

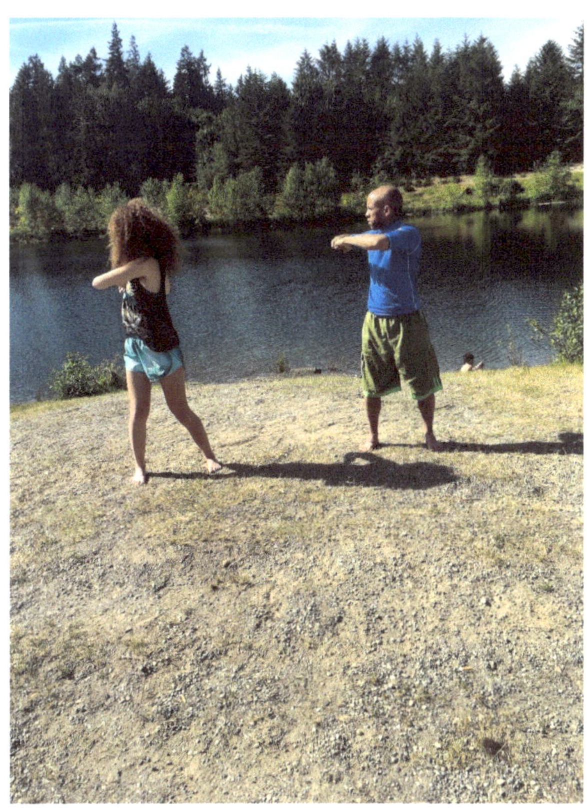

If your knees flex you are doing it wrong. We want our knees and thighs unmoving while our upper body swings back and forth from the hips up. Maintain proper breathing and proper balance.

Hip Rotations
Imagine you have a pole that runs straight down from the top of your head through your torso and down to the floor. Sink into Horse Stance. Remember proper breath and proper balance. Imagine only your hips are free from this pole. Now rotate your hips clockwise around the pole without moving anything other than your hips, allowing no wobble in your upper or lower body. (Belly Dancing lessons are great for this movement.)

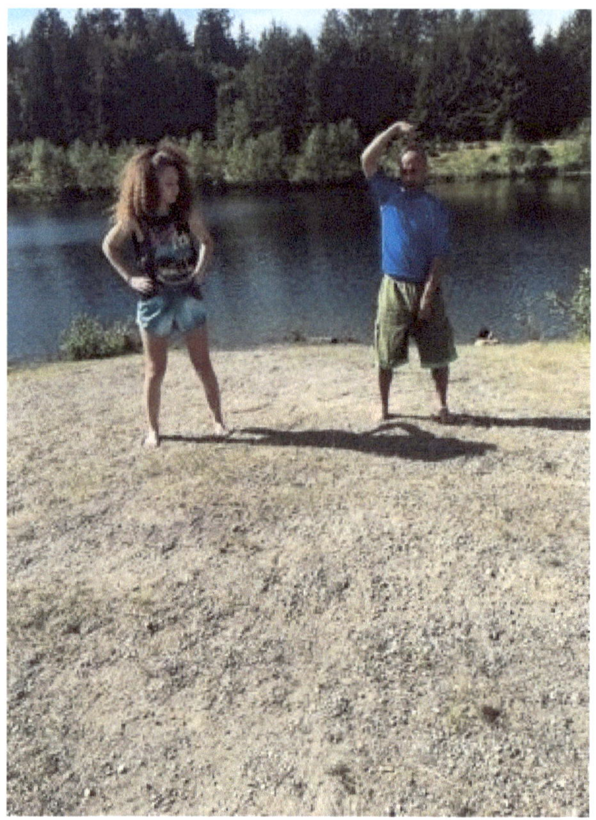

Rotating Knees

Rotate your knees toward each other. The goal is to keep the rest of the body still while rotating your knees. This may be hard at first and will get easier with time. Remember proper breathing and proper balance. Reverse direction.

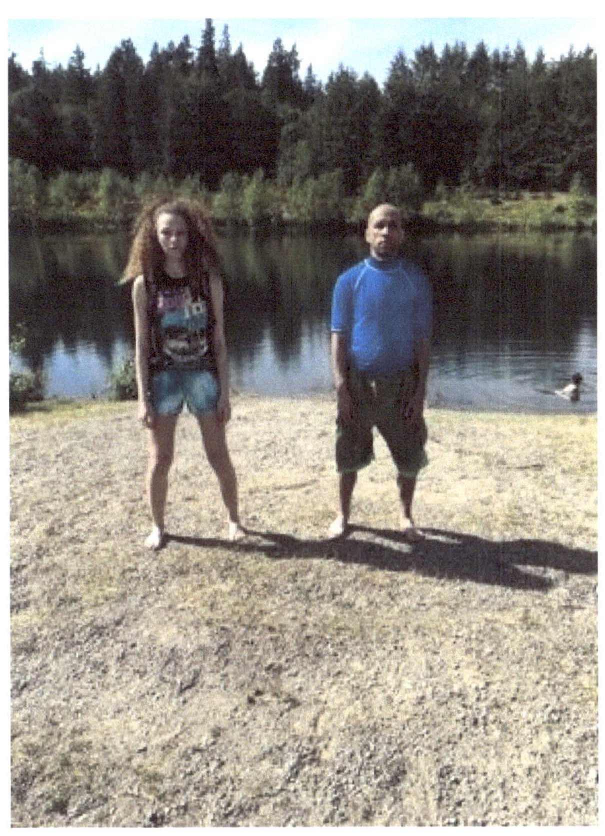

Digging Feet

Find your good Horse Stance. Get up on the balls of your feet. Rotate your body and feet slightly assuming a fighting stance. Find proper breathing and balance. Spread the toes on your back foot and begin rotating your ankle mashing the ball of your foot into mat. As you rotate your ankle, feel each toe flex, dig in and work each toe individually. Imagine an animal's foot ripping into to the ground. Reverse direction. Find Horse Stance. Switch Fighting Foot position. Repeat.

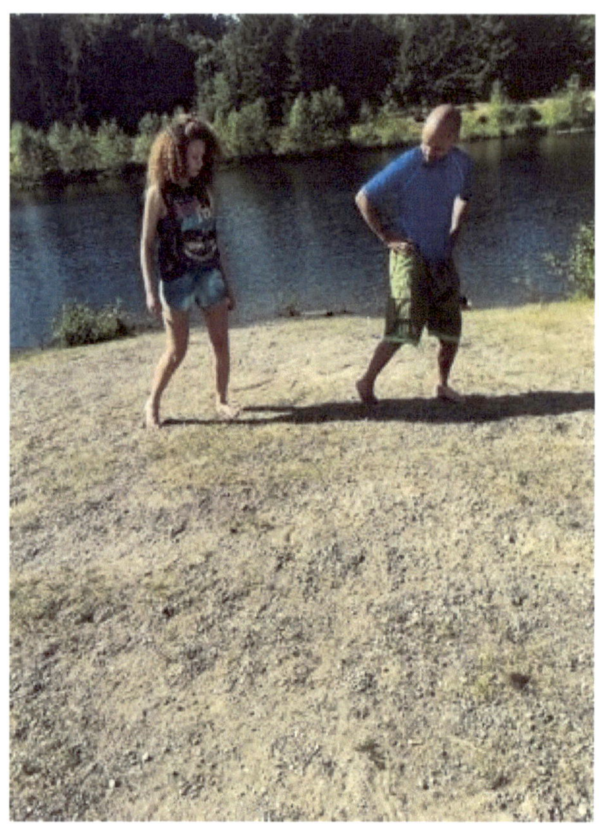

Stretch
We relax to extend the muscles, and. Little to no force is needed. You can hold each stretch for approx. 20 seconds

 Keeping Horse Stance throughout our stretches, maintaining proper breathing and proper balance.

 Place left hand across head and rest it flat on the right side of your head. Do not pull. Relax your neck Relax right arm to the floor and let the weight of your arm drag your neck toward the floor.
 Repeat on the other side.

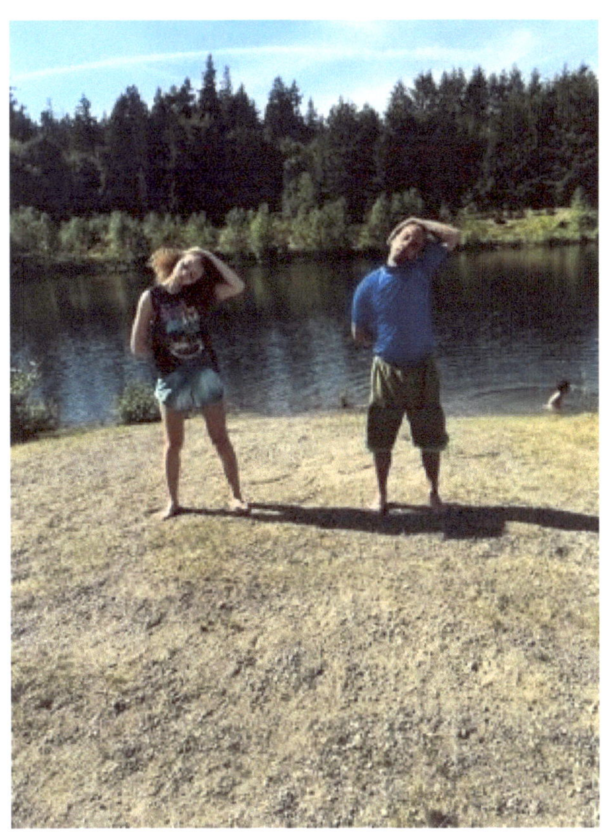

Wrap both hands around the back of your head. Pinch your elbows together. Rest your neck and relax your arms to the floor.

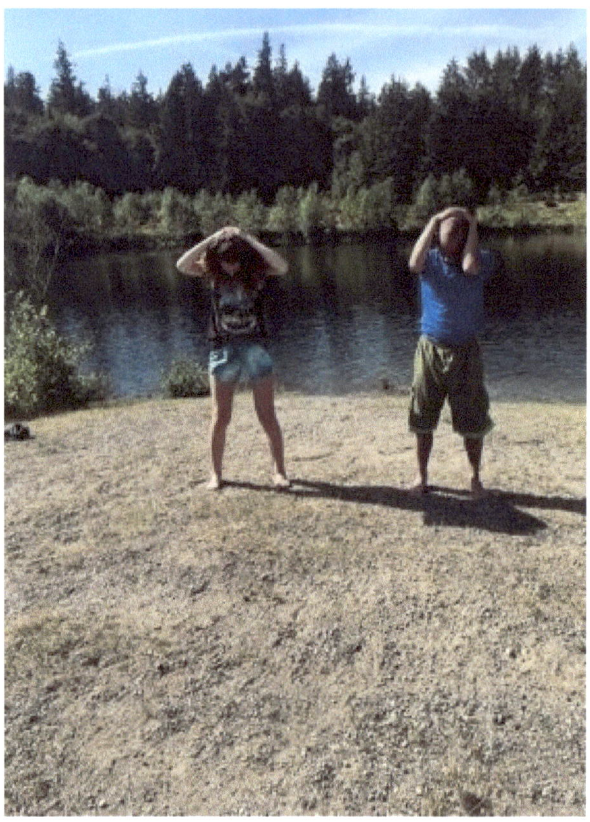

Cross your left arm across your chest to the opposite side.
Place right hand on left shoulder. Slowly slide your hand from your shoulder to your fingertips within 20 seconds.
 Repeat on the other side.

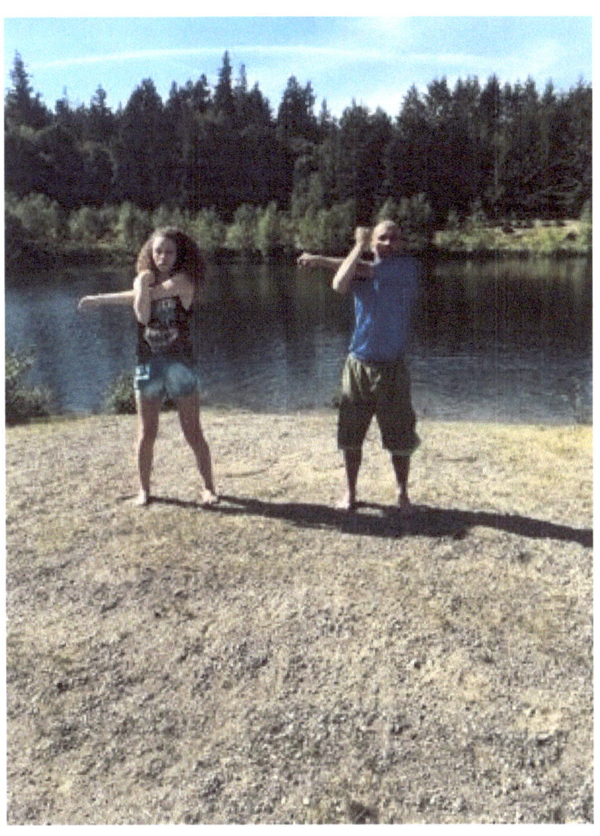

Place feet as near each other as you can while maintaining good balance. Raise your right hand directly above your head and relax your right hip as far out to the right as far as you can while maintaining proper breathing and proper balance. Let your raised hand relax to the floor. Let the hand on the hip relax deep into the hip.

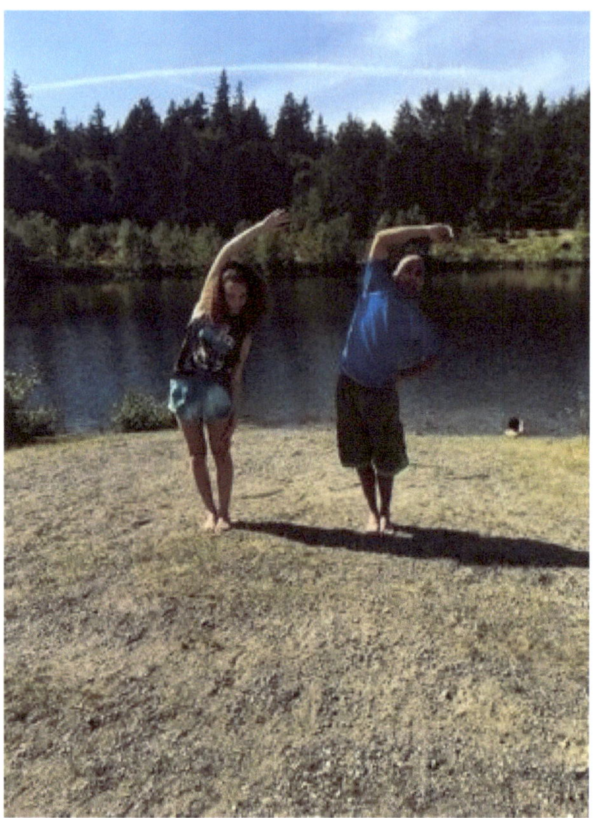

 Feel free to explore your stretch within a range of motion that keeps your balance. Repeat on the other side.
 As you gain balance, you will be able to bring your feet to touching and then to crossing.

 Stand on one foot. Bend your right foot to your right buttock. Use your right hand to grab your right foot and keep it pressed against your buttock. Do not pull or strain. Keep left knee soft just like regular Horse Stance. Find proper posture, proper breathing and proper balance. Place your left hand on your center line between your chest muscles to keep from wobbling. Tilt your hips forward and up.
 Repeat on the other side.

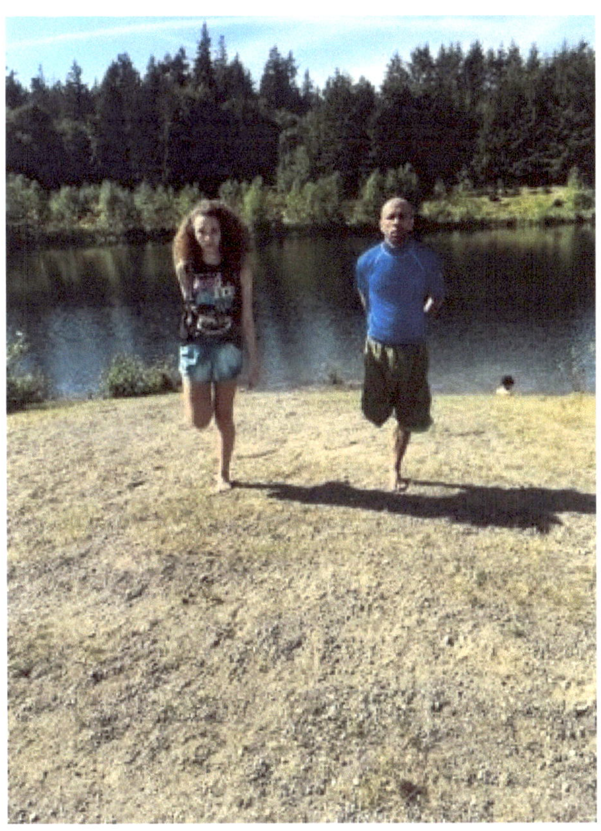

Find a proper Fat Horse Stance. Remember to maintain soft knees. Bend at the waist relaxing your upper body forward and breathing out, allowing your upper body to hang loosely. Remember proper breath and proper balance.

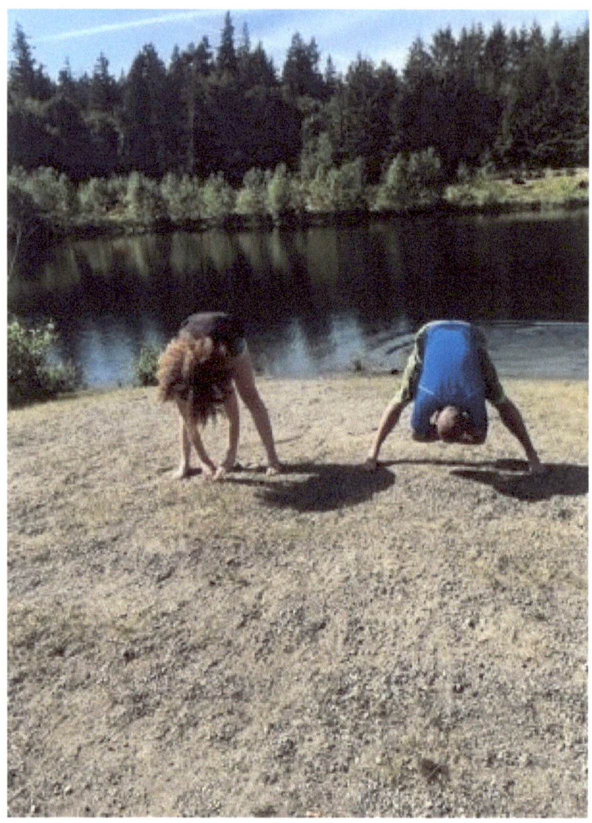

Assume Horse Stance. Place your hands at shoulder width in front of your feet. Walk your hands out to downward dog position.

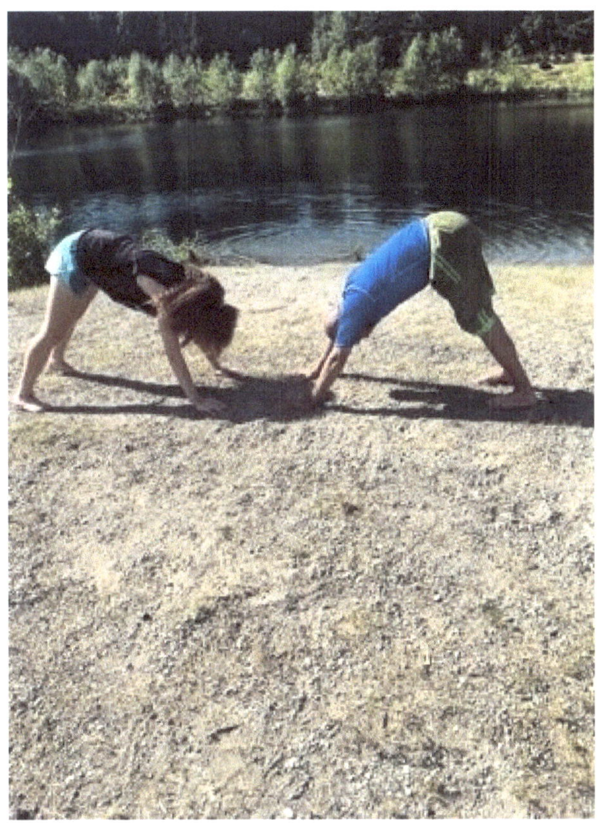

Relax your entire body with emphasis on relaxing your heals to the floor. Walk hands back and return to Horse Stance.

Simple Workout

This workout can be done individually or with a partner. With a partner we get larger rest periods, higher reps, more motivation and another eye toward gaining precision.

Try for 10 reps per movement alone or 20 reps per movement with a partner. Cycle through these movements until you reach 100 reps per movement.

10 Jumping Jacks

Remember breathing and balance point. Keep a steady rhythm. Stay on the balls of your feet. Start with a Skinny Horse Stance. Jump feet out to Fat Horse Stance. Return to Skinny Horse Stance. Make each rebound smooth. No slamming down. Stay on the balls of your feet and imagine they are spring loaded.

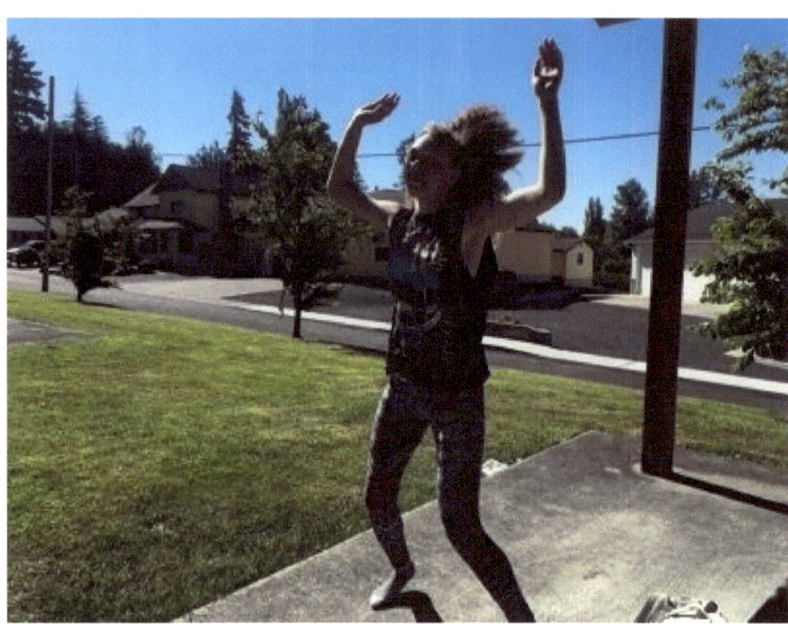

10 Push Ups

 Lay face down and flat Place each hand under matching shoulder Place toes shoulder width apart with legs full extended Keeping head, back, butt and heals in a straight line as you fully extend your arms pushing your chest away from the floor. Breathing and balance point is still important here. Lower your chest toward the floor, not all the way to the floor but close. It is perfectly fine to drop to your knees. Our goal is to keep going. If you have to stop and rest or stretch (at all), you're doing it wrong.

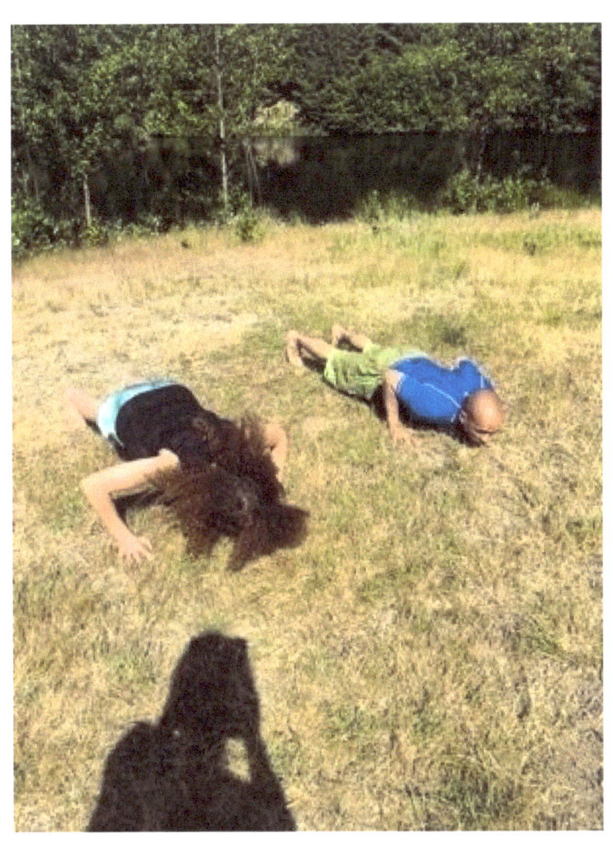

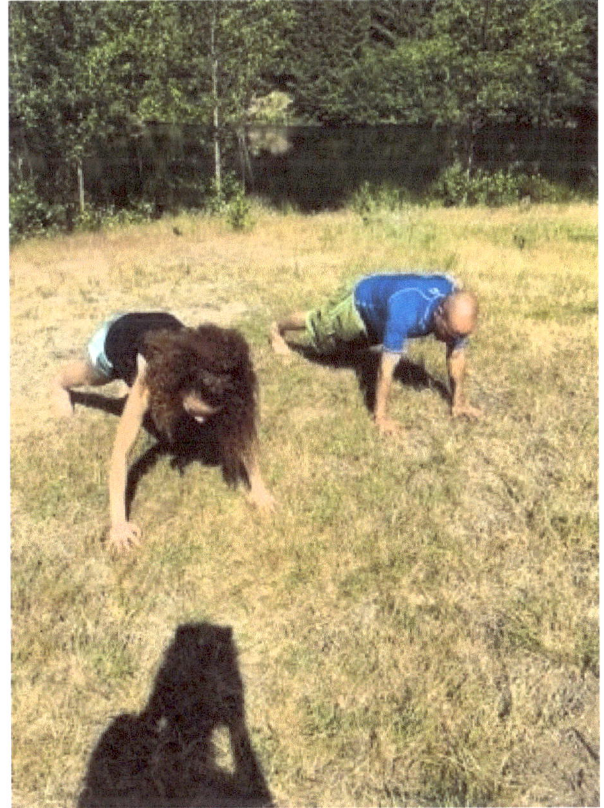

10 Crunches

Lay on your back with your feet shoulder width apart and 1 foot from your butt. Raise your chest toward your knees

You will feel a natural rebound and this is where you return your back to the floor If you have a partner, keep your feet together Have them place their knees next to each of your feet. Their chest can press against your shins and hold you knees. Breath and balance points are also important here.

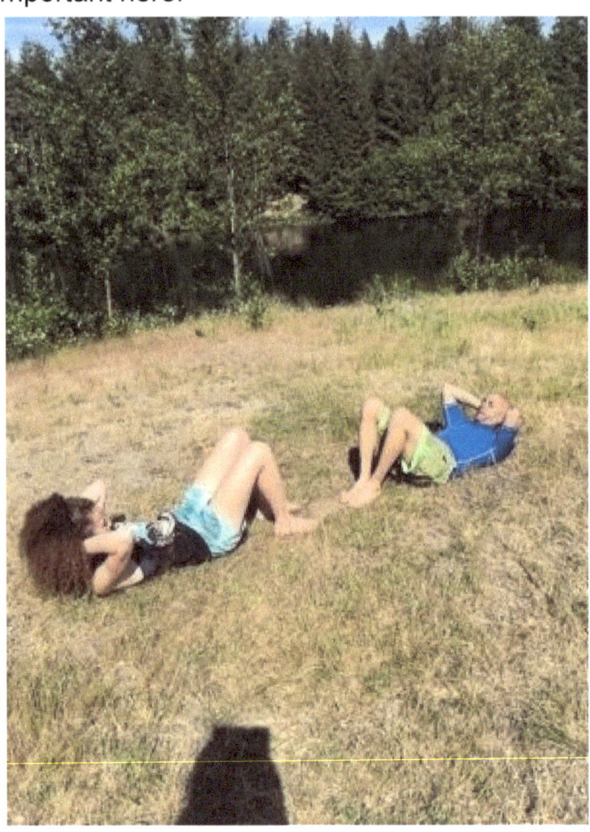

10 Squats

Stand with your feet shoulder width apart or slightly further apart Imagine sitting on a low chair Keep your back straight and your chin up Lower your butt toward the ground until your butt falls below chair seat height Return to standing Repeat Repeat this cycle until you reach 100 of each movement.

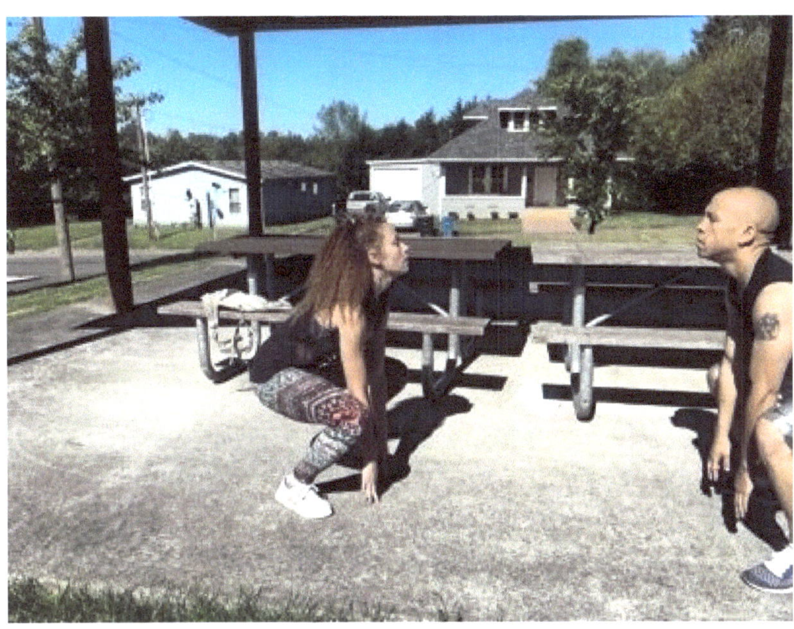

10 Chair dips

Place your hands, palms down and fingers forward with your butt directly in between. Butt should be resting on the edge of a structure one could comfortably sit on. Legs are extended fully or bent at knees. If your knees are bent, keep your feet shoulder width apart. Lower your butt towards the floor.

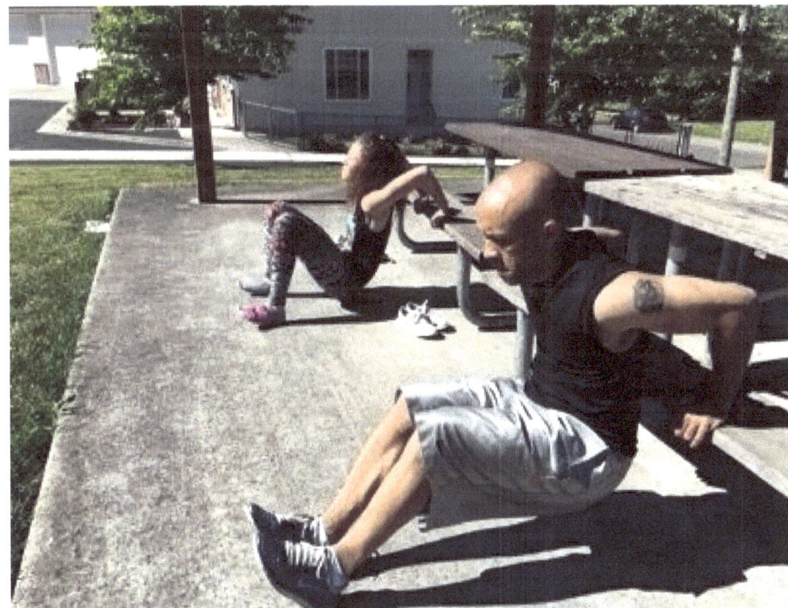

Remember proper breath and proper balance. Raise your butt back up as far as you can. Rest here is fine, to rest just sit on the edge of the structure.

As you go about your day practice letting small things go. You can apply this when banging your shin or stubbing your toe. If nothing is broken you can breathe, stay focused and quickly forget the irritation. This can be applied to mental irritation as well. As with all these practices, don't be afraid to start small.

Chapter 4

MENTAL DIET

Gain concrete definitions for the words and phrases you use and hear. A dictionary app works amazing. I use Merriam Webster Dictionary HD. This will help you sharpen your intent and realize others' intent for you.
Reference our Glossary Chapter as a start. We made the Glossary a Chapter to emphasize the practice of words toward mental diet.
Become more interested in the words and thoughts you use and how you use them. Become more aware of the words and thoughts other people use and how they use them. Add or subtract words and phrases from your vocabulary according to your intent. Abracadabra is an old word meaning "I create what I speak." The Bible says, "At first there was the word." Many religions and many practices emphasize the power of sound and or words. Now, I'm no religious man yet I believe the men who documented these principals were smart men, great thinkers, and great observers.

So, begin by cutting out phrases or words that detract from your intent. For instance, "FML" or , (Fuck My Life.), in text speak, is a phrase I cringe at every time and when I see people post it on social media. If at first there is the word, this person is creating what they speak then they are fucking their life and if I am in their life, I'm fucked.

It may be hard to just quit cold turkey, so here is a practice I developed for getting me closer. If I found myself saying I couldn't do something, I started adding the word YET.
I can't run that fast, YET. I can't say no YET. It works great. I suggested it to my nephew when he was trying to land a skateboard trick. He was telling me the
story of how he can't land this trick. I suggested he add YET. He said out loud that he couldn't land it YET and he landed it on his very next try not 5 seconds after changing the way he spoke about his intent. Yet is a powerful word, and can help you bridge that mental gap and begin eliminating words like CAN'T.

I have noticed in my own training and when training others, when we mess up, we tend to mess up again right away, and may even get stuck in a negative feedback. I fix this hiccup within myself by immediately moving on if I make a mistake. The mistake is only seen as a cue toward getting it right. If I think about the hiccup the hiccup repeats.

I have trained fighters and been around fighters, and I always suggest they stay away from people who come to them after a loss or injury repeating how it sucks. I encourage the fighters to concentrate on what they did right and what they did wrong, not on the emotion and not on how much it sucks. Other people's words have power too. If you are trying to focus on fixing things, and they are redirecting you toward sadness and woe, then you do not have the same intent, and you need to cut them out of the conversation or set clear boundaries beforehand as to how you wish to address your life. This can apply to anger, lust, sloth, greed and so on. Pay attention to how someone steers you with their words. Pay attention to where you steer yourself with your words.

Turn the TV off. You may think you're shutting down and resting when you plop down to watch TV but really you are just switching to a different modality that can run on high rev. We we can witness this when watching a scary movie, or one that makes us cry for sadness or compassion. Point is, you are being steered in a direction toward powerful emotions or instincts not of your own choosing, and this whittles away at your energy and ability to steer yourself.

Stressful things can go away, for instance, that end table you keep banging your toe on. How great would it be to wake up and not instantly bang your toe and consuming stress before consuming breakfast? Begin with small things and as you gain mental strength it will turn into big things. The big things will turn into huge things and so on.

Listen to music, comedy or a podcast that brings your energy up upon getting up and moving around. Having something going that gives us some pep while preparing breakfast, can set a precedent toward a more positive attitude toward food for that day and set a great mood.

Morning motivators:

Comedians that get me going
Pablo Francisco @pablo_francisco
Bill Burr @billburr
Joe Rogan @joerogan

Music that gets me going
Woodkid - Run Boy Run @woodkidmusic
Die Antwoord - Fatty Boom Boom (Heavy Metal Version) @dieantwoord
Biz Markie - Nobody Beats the Biz @officialbizmarkie

Podcasts that get me going
Daniele Bolelli, "History on Fire"
Inspire Nation @inspire7billion
The James Altucher Show @altucher

Chapter 5

PERSONAL INSTINCT

Obsessive/Perfectionist?

You used to see obsessiveness as a negative trait that only gets in the way and ruins progress in your mental and physical practices. You became engrossed in physical or mental practices to the extent that your mind and or body were left broken or burnt out. Now you are becoming obsessive about having the type of life that lends to your overall mental and physical well being. This will take time to fully sharpen, and with obsessive practice, goals can be achieved.

If you have family and friends that must have a portion of your time, be obsessive about taking time for them. Notice I said "taking time" not making time. Making time lends to the idea that a 25th hour must be manifested as if by magic. Taking time lends to a more empowering frame of mind where we have 24 hours and we will figure out how to use them. You're in control. You have time. Do not accept anything less than having time for the people and things you love.

Making your bed first thing and downing two glasses of water every morning should be easy and satisfying for you. You get to satisfy your obsessive compulsion immediately.

Satisfying these tendencies immediately should lend to a smoother transition into meditation. Obsession and focus can go hand in hand. Remember, great energy but little stress.

Obsessiveness is great for Horse Stance. Most flooring has lines or patterns that lend greatly to intentional foot placement. Place your feet on certain lines or patterns every time to satisfy your compulsion. Don't forget to notice how proper stance feels though and become obsessive about getting the feel right for those times you don't have a pattern to adhere to. The same applies for hand placement for Push Ups or Chair Dips. Going slow should be easy for an obsessive person, you want to get it right. Slowing down will lend to getting it right faster. And when your form starts breaking down, you can readily move on to another practice where good form is more easily achieved.

If you are obsessive, you will be paying very close attention so as to get it right. This mindset is perfect for stretching in my mind. We can really notice every muscle and tendon extending toward our goal. Again, be obsessive about foot placement, relaxation, proper breathing and proper balance.

Obsession toward rest is amazing. Pick a day, Sunday works for me. This is a practice that predates written history. Like your other obsessions, pick a rest day and do not break this practice. Do not cook, (fresh raw fruits and vegetables are perfect for this. Or even pre made meals,) do not clean, do not study, do not work. This all seems anti intuitive to our modern world but I guarantee the payoff in mental and physical progress is worth it. Rest is a practice that takes a lot of effort at first.

Keeping notes should be easy for you. Great notes and great note reviewing will allow you to more readily find the patterns in your daily practices that are not lending or are lending to your goals.

Hyperactive/Lacking attention

You used to think people couldn't stand being around you because you are too much. You used to think that you have to calm down to get anything done. But you have been practicing your mental diet and are now abstaining from hanging out with people who bum you out. You notice how only consuming good vibes concerning yourself has helped you begin to focus the tornado that is you. You have noticed that being fully yourself allows you to more readily accomplish mental and physical tasks. You pour yourself into individual people, places and things. Going crazy on tasks for an hour at a time. Go until you can't go any more at one thing, then switch to another thing. Finding something to do all day every day is fun and you get to learn a ridiculous amount of things in a short amount of time.

You don't have to make time because you're able to get where you gotta go fast. You will be able to drop the thing you aren't really making progress on right now and move forward in another thing and hop back to the last thing when the mood comes back and the proper tools have been attained. You have time for friends who need help moving, if a pickup game of Basketball breaks out, Kids need to be lead away from the TV and toward a game of tag? That's you. You are the life of the party.

Waking up making your bed and drinking two tall glasses of water first thing will immediately satisfy that need you have to get a solid grasp on your day. The water will rev up your body system and be a major driver toward the high energy day you are in for.

Satisfying that need to have a solid grasp on your day will lend to a smoother transition into meditation. You only need to meditate for a short time which is perfect for you. You can meditate on focus or energy depending on your needs that day.

Hyperactivity is great for getting things done like right now! No need to wait. With precision and enthusiasm you can get things done fast and have the energy to continue lengthy tasks or begin new ones after completing others. Hyperactivity lends to testing proper balance and breathing non stop. With proper breathing and balance your energy has multiplied and you're not crashing into things and people any more. Less mental and physical friction is what allows you to harness excessive energy.

Rest is important and may be a task at first. The ability to rest can be it's own battle and maybe that challenge will be what drives you. Lively podcasts are how I began handling my hyperactivity on rest days initially. I used my obsessiveness to chip away at that so now I can just chill on those days. Lively podcasts and books get me pumped and that is not my goal on rest day.

Keeping notes should be easy for you. It gives you something to do and is a great outlet for your energy. You can begin to see who and what drags you down and what keeps your blood pumping.

Over Analytical?

You used to think that you overthink things and struggled between who you thought you were and the idea that immediate action is what is needed. You spent all of your time planning to the extent that you had no time and or energy to act on your conclusions. Now you are noticing how analyzing data in real time is extremely satisfying and has magnified your analytical abilities. Analyzing results based on action has only served to satisfy your need for data. This will take time to fully grasp and the proof will be in the pudding.

You have been paying closer attention to your own motivations and emotions in real time and this has helped you understand your relationships instead of analyzing them. This is drawing people to you rather than pushing them away or having the time spent with them drag everyone down.

Making your bed first thing in the morning and drinking two tall glasses of water can immediately be analyzed by noticing how it truly does set precedent for the day. This observation can be applied to many things throughout your life.

Satisfying this tendency should allow an easy transition into meditation. This is another practice that can be tracked in real time and documented for further evaluation later.

An analytical mind is as great for physical practice as it is for mental. Keen observation of proper breathing and proper balance can only serve to improve overall fitness. It is ok to take it slow, paying attention to every sensation and thought. Just remember that to gather data properly one must gather experience.

An analytical mind can readily notice improved mental and physical states. Make sure that you are not pouring over or taking notes on rest day or your data will be skewed and lack precision. Rest on rest day, observe the results, document the next day.

Of course taking notes is very satisfying for the analytical mind and cannot help but make the transition to your desired outcome smoother.

GLOSSARY

fit·ness\\ˈfit-nəs\

noun

1 : the quality or state of being fit

2 : the capacity of an organism to survive and transmit its genotype to reproductive offspring as compared to competing organisms; also : the contribution of an allele or genotype to the gene pool of subsequent generations as compared to that of other alleles or genotypes

Examples

a gymnastics program promoting fitness and agility in school-aged children

I have to question the fitness of wearing a bright red dress to a funeral.

2fit adjective

: proper or acceptable : morally or socially correct

: suitable for a specified purpose

: physically healthy and strong

Full Definition

1 a (1) : adapted to an end or design : suitable by nature or by art (2) : adapted to the environment so as to be capable of surviving

b : acceptable from a particular viewpoint (as of competence or morality) : proper <a movie fit for the whole family>

2 a : put into a suitable state : made ready <get the house fit for company>

b : being in such a state as to be or seem ready to do or suffer something <fair fit to cry I was — Bryan MacMahon> <laughing fit to burst>

3 : sound physically and mentally : healthy

fat\\ˈfat\

adjective

: having a lot of extra flesh on your body : having a lot of body fat

: having a full, rounded form

: unusually wide or thick

Full Definition

1 : notable for having an unusual amount of fat:

a : plump

b : obese

c of a meat animal : fattened for market

d of food : oily, greasy

2 a : well filled out : thick, big <a fat book>

b : full in tone and quality : rich <a gorgeous fat bass voice — Irish Digest>

c : well stocked <a fat larder>

d : prosperous, wealthy <grew fat on the war — Time>

e : being substantial and impressive <a fat bank account>

3 a : richly rewarding or profitable <a fat part in a movie> <a fat contract>

b : practically nonexistent <a fat chance>

4 : productive, fertile <a fat year for crops>
5 : stupid, foolish
6 : being swollen <got a fat lip from the fight>
7 of a baseball pitch : easy to hit

health\ˈhelth also ˈheltth\
noun
: the condition of being well or free from disease
: the overall condition of someone's body or mind
: the condition or state of something
Full Definition
Usage: often attributive
1 a : the condition of being sound in body, mind, or spirit; especially : freedom from physical disease or pain
b : the general condition of the body <in poor health> <enjoys good health>
2 a : flourishing condition : well-being <defending the health of the beloved oceans — Peter Wilkinson>
b : general condition or state <poor economic health>
3 : a toast to someone's health or prosperity

med·i·cine\ˈme-də-sən, British usually ˈmed-sən\
noun
: a substance that is used in treating disease or relieving pain and that is usually in the form of a pill or a liquid
: the science that deals with preventing, curing, and treating diseases
Full Definition
1 a : a substance or preparation used in treating disease
b : something that affects well-being
2 a : the science and art dealing with the maintenance of health and the prevention, alleviation, or cure of disease
b : the branch of medicine concerned with the nonsurgical treatment of disease
3 : a substance (as a drug or potion) used to treat something other than disease
4 : an object held in traditional American Indian belief to give control over natural or magical forces; also : magical power or a magical rite

stress\ˈstres\
noun
: a state of mental tension and worry caused by problems in your life, work, etc.
: something that causes strong feelings of worry or anxiety
: physical force or pressure
Full Definition
1 : constraining force or influence: as
a : a force exerted when one body or body part presses on, pulls on, pushes against, or tends to

compress or twist another body or body part; especially : the intensity of this mutual force commonly expressed in pounds per square inch
b : the deformation caused in a body by such a force
c : a physical, chemical, or emotional factor that causes bodily or mental tension and may be a factor in disease causation
d : a state resulting from a stress; especially : one of bodily or mental tension resulting from factors that tend to alter an existent equilibrium <job-related stress>
e : strain, pressure <the environment is under stress to the point of collapse — Joseph Shoben>
2 : emphasis, weight <lay stress on a point>
3 archaic : intense effort or exertion
4 : intensity of utterance given to a speech sound, syllable, or word producing relative loudness
5 a : relative force or prominence of sound in verse
b : a syllable having relative force or prominence
6 : accent 6a

re·laxed\ri-ˈlakst\
adjective
: calm and free from stress, worry, or anxiety : not worried or tense
: informal and comfortable
: not strict or carefully controlled
Full Definition
1 : freed from or lacking in precision or stringency
2 : set or being at rest or at ease
3 : easy of manner : informal
4 : somewhat loose-fitting and usually casual in style <relaxed jeans>

peace\ˈpēs\
noun
: a state in which there is no war or fighting
: an agreement to end a war
: a period of time when there is no war or fighting
Full Definition
1 : a state of tranquillity or quiet: as
a : freedom from civil disturbance
b : a state of security or order within a community provided for by law or custom <a breach of the peace>
2 : freedom from disquieting or oppressive thoughts or emotions
3 : harmony in personal relations
4 a : a state or period of mutual concord between governments
b : a pact or agreement to end hostilities between those who have been at war or in a state of enmity
5 —used interjectionally to ask for silence or calm or as a greeting or farewell
at peace : in a state of concord or tranquillity

bal·ance\ˈba-lən(t)s\
noun
: the state of having your weight spread equally so that you do not fall
: the ability to move or to remain in a position without losing control or falling
: a state in which different things occur in equal or proper amounts or have an equal or proper
amount of importance
Full Definition
1 : an instrument for weighing: as
a : a beam that is supported freely in the center and has two pans of equal weight suspended
from its ends
b : a device that uses the elasticity of a spiral spring for measuring weight or force
2 : a means of judging or deciding
3 : a counterbalancing weight, force, or influence
4 : an oscillating wheel operating with a hairspring to regulate the movement of a timepiece
5 a : stability produced by even distribution of weight on each side of the vertical axis
b : equipoise between contrasting, opposing, or interacting elements
c : equality between the totals of the two sides of an account
6 a : an aesthetically pleasing integration of elements
b : the juxtaposition in writing of syntactically parallel constructions containing similar or
contrasting ideas
7 a : physical equilibrium
b : the ability to retain one's balance
8 a : weight or force of one side in excess of another
b : something left over : remainder
c : an amount in excess especially on the credit side of an account
9 : mental and emotional steadiness

knowl·edge\ˈnä-lij\
noun
: information, understanding, or skill that you get from experience or education
: awareness of something : the state of being aware of something
Full Definition
1 obsolete : cognizance
2 a (1) : the fact or condition of knowing something with familiarity gained through experience or
association (2) : acquaintance with or understanding of a science, art, or technique
b (1) : the fact or condition of being aware of something (2) : the range of one's information or
understanding <answered to the best of my knowledge>
c : the circumstance or condition of apprehending truth or fact through reasoning : cognition
d : the fact or condition of having information or of being learned <a person of unusual
knowledge>
3 archaic : sexual intercourse
4 a : the sum of what is known : the body of truth, information, and principles acquired by

humankind
b archaic : a branch of learning

in·sight\ˈin-ˌsīt\
noun
: the ability to understand people and situations in a very clear way
: an understanding of the true nature of something
Full Definition
1 : the power or act of seeing into a situation : penetration
2 : the act or result of apprehending the inner nature of things or of seeing intuitively

any·thing\-ˌthiŋ\
pronoun
: a thing of any kind
Full Definition
: any thing whatever : any such thing

will·pow·er\ˈwil-ˌpau̇(-ə)r\
noun
: the ability to control yourself : strong determination that allows you to do something difficult
(such as to lose weight or quit smoking)
Full Definition
: energetic determination

cal·o·rie
noun
: a unit of heat used to indicate the amount of energy that foods will produce in the human body
Full Definition
1 a : the amount of heat required at a pressure of one atmosphere to raise the temperature of
one gram of water one degree Celsius that is equal to about 4.19 joules — abbreviation cal
—called also gram calorie, small calorie
b : the amount of heat required to raise the temperature of one kilogram of water one degree
Celsius : 1000 gram calories or 3.968 Btu — abbreviation Cal —called also large calorie
2 a : a unit equivalent to the large calorie expressing heat-producing or energy-producing value
in food when oxidized in the body
b : an amount of food having an energy-producing value of one large calorie

sta·bil·i·ty\stə-ˈbi-lə-tē\
noun
: the quality or state of something that is not easily changed or likely to change
: the quality or state of something that is not easily moved
: the quality or state of someone who is emotionally or mentally healthy
Full Definition

1 : the quality, state, or degree of being stable: as
a : the strength to stand or endure : firmness
b : the property of a body that causes it when disturbed from a condition of equilibrium or steady motion to develop forces or moments that restore the original condition
c : resistance to chemical change or to physical disintegration
2 : residence for life in one monastery

strength\\ˈstreŋ(k)th, ˈstren(t)th\
noun
: the quality or state of being physically strong
: the ability to resist being moved or broken by a force
: the quality that allows someone to deal with problems in a determined and effective way
Full Definition
1 : the quality or state of being strong : capacity for exertion or endurance
2 : power to resist force : solidity, toughness
3 : power of resisting attack : impregnability
4 a : legal, logical, or moral force
b : a strong attribute or inherent asset <the strengths and the weaknesses of the book are evident>
5 a : degree of potency of effect or of concentration <chili peppers in varying strengths>
b : intensity of light, color, sound, or odor
c : vigor of expression
6 : force as measured in numbers : effective numbers of any body or organization <an army at full strength>
7 : one regarded as embodying or affording force or firmness : support <you are my love and my strength>
8 : maintenance of or a rising tendency in a price level : firmness of prices <the strength of the dollar>
9 : basis — used in the phrase on the strength of

di·et\ˈdī-ət\
noun
1 a : food and drink regularly provided or consumed
b : habitual nourishment
c : the kind and amount of food prescribed for a person or animal for a special reason
d : a regimen of eating and drinking sparingly so as to reduce one's weight <going on a diet>
2 : something provided or experienced repeatedly <a diet of Broadway shows and nightclubs — Frederick Wyatt>

dis·ease\di-ˈzēz\
noun
: an illness that affects a person, animal, or plant : a condition that prevents the body or mind from working normally

: a problem that a person, group, organization, or society has and cannot stop
Full Definition
1 obsolete : trouble
2 : a condition of the living animal or plant body or of one of its parts that impairs normal
functioning and is typically manifested by distinguishing signs and symptoms : sickness, malady
3 : a harmful development (as in a social institution)

truth\ˈtrüth\
noun
: the real facts about something : the things that are true
: the quality or state of being true
: a statement or idea that is true or accepted as true
Full Definition
1 a archaic : fidelity, constancy
b : sincerity in action, character, and utterance
2 a (1) : the state of being the case : fact (2) : the body of real things, events, and facts :
actuality (3) often capitalized : a transcendent fundamental or spiritual reality
b : a judgment, proposition, or idea that is true or accepted as true <truths of thermodynamics>
c : the body of true statements and propositions
3 a : the property (as of a statement) of being in accord with fact or reality
b chiefly British : true 2
c : fidelity to an original or to a standard
4 capitalized Christian Science : god

self–con·trol\-kən-ˈtrōl\
noun
: control over your feelings or actions
Full Definition
: restraint exercised over one's own impulses, emotions, or desires

rest\ˈrest\
noun
1 : repose, sleep; specifically : a bodily state characterized by minimal functional and metabolic
activities
2 a : freedom from activity or labor
b : a state of motionlessness or inactivity
c : the repose of death
3 : a place for resting or lodging
4 : peace of mind or spirit
5 a (1) : a rhythmic silence in music (2) : a character representing such a silence
b : a brief pause in reading
6 : something used for support
at rest

1 : resting or reposing especially in sleep or death
2 : quiescent, motionless
3 : free of anxieties

in·spi·ra·tion\ˌin(t)-spə-ˈrā-shən, -(ˌ)spi-\
noun
: something that makes someone want to do something or that gives someone an idea about what to do or create : a force or influence that inspires someone
: a person, place, experience, etc., that makes someone want to do or create something
: a good idea
Full Definition
1 a : a divine influence or action on a person believed to qualify him or her to receive and communicate sacred revelation
b : the action or power of moving the intellect or emotions
c : the act of influencing or suggesting opinions
2 : the act of drawing in; specifically : the drawing of air into the lungs
3 a : the quality or state of being inspired
b : something that is inspired <a scheme that was pure inspiration>
4 : an inspiring agent or influence

mo·ti·va·tion\ˌmō-tə-ˈvā-shən\
noun
: the act or process of giving someone a reason for doing something : the act or process of motivating someone
: the condition of being eager to act or work : the condition of being motivated
: a force or influence that causes someone to do something
Full Definition
1 a : the act or process of motivating
b : the condition of being motivated
2 : a motivating force, stimulus, or influence : incentive, drive

fore·sight\ˈfȯr-ˌsīt\
noun
: the ability to see what will or might happen in the future
Full Definition
1 : an act or the power of foreseeing : prescience
2 : provident care : prudence <had the foresight to invest his money wisely>
3 : an act of looking forward; also : a view forward

cause\ˈkȯz\
noun
: something or someone that produces an effect, result, or condition : something or someone that makes something happen or exist

: a reason for doing or feeling something
: something (such as an organization, belief, idea, or goal) that a group or people support or fight for
Full Definition
1 a : a reason for an action or condition : motive
b : something that brings about an effect or a result
c : a person or thing that is the occasion of an action or state; especially : an agent that brings something about
d : sufficient reason <discharged for cause>
2 a : a ground of legal action
b : case
3 : a matter or question to be decided
4 a : a principle or movement militantly defended or supported
b : a charitable undertaking <for a good cause>

ef·fect\i-ˈfekt, e-, ē-, ə-\
noun
: a change that results when something is done or happens : an event, condition, or state of affairs that is produced by a cause
: a particular feeling or mood created by something
: an image or a sound that is created in television, radio, or movies to imitate something real
Full Definition
1 a : purport, intent
b : basic meaning : essence
2 : something that inevitably follows an antecedent (as a cause or agent)
3 : an outward sign : appearance
4 : accomplishment, fulfillment
5 : power to bring about a result : influence <the content itself of television…is therefore less important than its effect — Current Biography>
6 plural : movable property : goods <personal effects>
7 a : a distinctive impression <the color gives the effect of being warm>
b : the creation of a desired impression <her tears were purely for effect>
c (1) : something designed to produce a distinctive or desired impression — usually used in plural (2) plural : special effects
8 : the quality or state of being operative : operation <the law goes into effect next week>

prin·ci·ple\ˈprin(t)-s(ə-)pəl, -sə-bəl\
noun
: a moral rule or belief that helps you know what is right and wrong and that influences your actions
: a basic truth or theory : an idea that forms the basis of something
: a law or fact of nature that explains how something works or why something happens
Full Definition

1 a : a comprehensive and fundamental law, doctrine, or assumption
b (1) : a rule or code of conduct (2) : habitual devotion to right principles <a man of principle>
c : the laws or facts of nature underlying the working of an artificial device
2 : a primary source : origin
3 a : an underlying faculty or endowment <such principles of human nature as greed and curiosity>
b : an ingredient (as a chemical) that exhibits or imparts a characteristic quality
4 capitalized Christian Science : a divine principle : god

will·pow·er\ˈwil-ˌpau̇(-ə)r\
noun
: the ability to control yourself : strong determination that allows you to do something difficult (such as to lose weight or quit smoking)
Full Definition
: energetic determination

sick·ness\ˈsik-nəs\
noun
: unhealthy condition of body or mind : the state of being sick
: a specific type of disease or illness
: the feeling you have in your stomach when you think you are going to vomit
Full Definition
1 a : ill health : illness
b : a disordered, weakened, or unsound condition
2 : a specific disease
3 : nausea, queasiness

heal\ˈhēl\
: to become healthy or well again
: to make (someone or something) healthy or well again
Full Definition
transitive verb
1 a : to make sound or whole <heal a wound>
b : to restore to health
2 a : to cause (an undesirable condition) to be overcome : mend <the troubles…had not been forgotten, but they had been healed — William Power>
b : to patch up (a breach or division) <heal a breach between friends>
3 : to restore to original purity or integrity <healed of sin>
intransitive verb
: to return to a sound state

hon·es·ty\ˈä-nəs-tē\
noun

: the quality of being fair and truthful : the quality of being honest
Full Definition
1 obsolete : chastity
2 a : fairness and straightforwardness of conduct
b : adherence to the facts : sincerity
3 : any of a genus (Lunaria) of European herbs of the mustard family with toothed leaves and flat disk-shaped siliques

en·er·gy\ˈe-nər-jē\
noun
: ability to be active : the physical or mental strength that allows you to do things
: natural enthusiasm and effort
: usable power that comes from heat, electricity, etc.
Full Definition
1 a : dynamic quality <narrative energy>
b : the capacity of acting or being active <intellectual energy>
c : a usually positive spiritual force <the energy flowing through all people>
2 : vigorous exertion of power : effort <investing time and energy>
3 : a fundamental entity of nature that is transferred between parts of a system in the production of physical change within the system and usually regarded as the capacity for doing work
4 : usable power (as heat or electricity); also : the resources for producing such power

teach·er\ˈtē-chər\
noun
: a person or thing that teaches something ; especially : a person whose job is to teach students about certain subjects
Full Definition
1 : one that teaches; especially : one whose occupation is to instruct
2 : a Mormon ranking above a deacon in the Aaronic priesthood

stu·dent\ˈstü-dənt, ˈstyü-, chiefly Southern -dənt\
noun
: a person who attends a school, college, or university
: a person who studies something
Full Definition
Usage: often attributive
1 : scholar, learner; especially : one who attends a school
2 : one who studies : an attentive and systematic observer <a student of politics>

Share:
to have or use (something) with others
of two or more people : to divide (something) into parts and each take or use a part
: to let someone else have or use a part of (something that belongs to you)

Full Definition
transitive verb
1 : to divide and distribute in shares : apportion — usually used with out <shared out the land among his heirs>
2 a : to partake of, use, experience, occupy, or enjoy with others
b : to have in common <they share a passion for opera>
3 : to grant or give a share in — often used with with <shared the last of her water with us>
4 : to tell (as thoughts, feelings, or experiences) to others — often used with with

short·cut\'short-ˌkət also -'kət\
noun
: a shorter, quicker, or easier way to get to a place
: a quicker or easier way to do something
Full Definition
1 : a route more direct than the one ordinarily taken
2 : a method or means of doing something more directly and quickly than and often not so thoroughly as by ordinary procedure <a shortcut to success>

do·ing\'dü-iŋ\
noun
: the act of making something happen through your own action
: things that someone does : things that happen
Full Definition
1 : the act of performing or executing : action <that will take a great deal of doing>
2 plural
a : things that are done or that occur : goings-on <everyday doings>
b : social activities

re·spect\ri-'spekt\
noun
: a feeling of admiring someone or something that is good, valuable, important, etc.
: a feeling or understanding that someone or something is important, serious, etc., and should be treated in an appropriate way
: a particular way of thinking about or looking at something
Full Definition
1 : a relation or reference to a particular thing or situation <remarks having respect to an earlier plan>
2 : an act of giving particular attention : consideration
3 a : high or special regard : esteem
b : the quality or state of being esteemed
c plural : expressions of high or special regard or deference <paid our respects>
4 : particular, detail <a good plan in some respects>

in respect of chiefly British : with respect to : concerning
in respect to : with respect to : concerning
with respect to : with reference to : in relation to

rest\ˈrest\
noun
1 : repose, sleep; specifically : a bodily state characterized by minimal functional and metabolic
activities
2 a : freedom from activity or labor
b : a state of motionlessness or inactivity
c : the repose of death
3 : a place for resting or lodging
4 : peace of mind or spirit
5 a (1) : a rhythmic silence in music (2) : a character representing such a silence
b : a brief pause in reading
6 : something used for support
at rest
1 : resting or reposing especially in sleep or death
2 : quiescent, motionless
3 : free of anxieties

ob·ses·sive\äb-ˈse-siv, əb-\
adjective
: thinking about something or someone too much or in a way that is not normal : having an
obsession : showing or relating to an obsession
Full Definition
1 a : tending to cause obsession
b : excessive often to an unreasonable degree
2 : of, relating to, or characterized by obsession : deriving from obsession

hy·per·ac·tive\ˌhī-pər-ˈak-tiv\
adjective
: extremely active or too active
Full Definition
1 : affected with or exhibiting hyperactivity; broadly : more active than is usual or desirable
2 : intricately or elaborately designed or detailed

*en·dure\in-ˈdur, -ˈdyur, en-\
: to continue to exist in the same state or condition
: to experience (pain or suffering) for a long time
: to deal with or accept (something unpleasant)

Full Definition
transitive verb
1 : to undergo (as a hardship) especially without giving in : suffer <endured great pain>
2 : to regard with acceptance or tolerance <could not endure noisy children>
intransitive verb
1 : to continue in the same state : last <the style endured for centuries>
2 : to remain firm under suffering or misfortune without yielding <though it is difficult, we must endure>

*hope\ˈhōp\
: to want something to happen or be true and think that it could happen or be true
Full Definition
intransitive verb
1 : to cherish a desire with anticipation <hopes for a promotion>
2 archaic : trust
transitive verb
1 : to desire with expectation of obtainment
2 : to expect with confidence : trust